LIFTING SPIRITS AND HEALING HEARTS

Family and Friends Ultimate Guide to Breast Cancer Support

by

Dr. Kristen Rea

Copyright © by Dr. Kristen Rea 2023.

TABLE OF CONTENT

Introduction

Understanding the Importance of Support

In the journey through breast cancer, the presence of a strong and compassionate support network can make an immense difference. The emotional and physical challenges that individuals facing breast cancer encounter can be overwhelming and the role of family, friends, and caregivers in providing unwavering support cannot be understated.

Support goes beyond mere assistance with tasks; it is the foundation upon which emotional well-being and resilience are built. When someone receives a breast cancer diagnosis, the shock and uncertainty can be paralyzing. It is during these moments that a network of understanding and caring individuals can help alleviate the weight of the burden.

Emotional Stability: The emotional turmoil that accompanies a breast cancer diagnosis can lead to feelings of isolation, fear, and anxiety. The presence of loved ones who offer a listening ear, a shoulder to cry on, or even just a warm hug can provide a sense of comfort and emotional stability. Knowing that one is not alone in their journey can foster hope and positivity.

Shared Burden: Breast cancer not only affects the individual diagnosed but also ripples through the lives of family members and close friends. Being a part of a support network allows loved ones to share in the burden, offering practical help and reassurance that they are in this together.

Navigating the Unknown: The world of medical treatments, procedures, and terminologies can be confusing and overwhelming for someone facing breast cancer. Having someone by their side who can provide information, ask questions during medical appointments, and ensure that all options are explored helps the patient make informed decisions.

Boosting Resilience: Studies have shown that those with a strong support system often demonstrate higher levels of resilience and coping skills. The encouragement, love, and reassurance provided by friends and family can enhance the patient's ability to overcome challenges and setbacks.

Advocacy and Empowerment: Supportive individuals can act as advocates, ensuring that the patient's voice is heard in medical decisions and treatment plans. This empowerment not only fosters a sense of control but also contributes to the patient's overall well-being.

Encouraging Communication: Open and honest communication between patients, caregivers, and loved ones is crucial. A strong support network encourages conversations about fears, hopes, and concerns, fostering an environment of understanding and trust.

In conclusion, understanding the importance of support in the breast cancer journey is essential for patients, caregivers, and loved ones alike. The bonds forged through compassion, empathy, and shared experiences can provide a lifeline of strength, comfort, and encouragement. By standing together, everyone involved can contribute to lifting spirits and healing hearts, making the path through breast cancer a little less daunting.

How This Book Can Help

Navigating the complexities of breast cancer can be a challenging and overwhelming experience for patients, as well as their families and friends. "Lifting Spirits, Healing Hearts: Family and Friend's Guide to Breast Cancer Support" aims to provide a comprehensive resource that offers guidance, understanding, and practical advice to those who find themselves in this journey of support.

Comprehensive Information: This book serves as a comprehensive guide, covering a wide range of topics related to breast cancer support. From understanding the different types of breast cancer and treatment options to offering insights into emotional resilience and self-care, this book covers it all. Readers can expect to find accurate, reliable information that helps them better understand the journey ahead.

Support Roles Clarified: One of the primary focuses of this book is to help family members and friends understand their roles in providing support. Clear guidance is provided on how to effectively communicate, offer practical help, and provide emotional support during various stages of the breast cancer journey.

Empathetic Guidance: Every chapter of the book is crafted with empathy and understanding. It acknowledges the emotional challenges faced by patients and caregivers and offers guidance on how to address these challenges with sensitivity and compassion. By offering insights into the emotional rollercoaster of breast cancer, the book helps caregivers and loved ones provide meaningful support.

Practical Strategies: "Lifting Spirits, Healing Hearts" goes beyond theory by offering practical strategies for supporting patients. It provides tips on assisting with daily activities, managing medical appointments, and creating a supportive environment. The book also includes advice on self-care for caregivers, ensuring that those providing support also prioritize their well-being.

Real-Life Stories: The book features stories from breast cancer survivors, patients, and caregivers. These personal narratives offer readers a glimpse into the real-world experiences of individuals who have faced breast cancer. These stories provide inspiration, encouragement, and relatable insights for both patients and their support network.

Resources and Further Assistance: Recognizing that every journey is unique, the book includes a comprehensive list of resources. Readers can find information on support groups, online communities, professional help, and additional reading materials. This ensures that readers have access to ongoing assistance beyond the pages of the book.

In essence, "Lifting Spirits, Healing Hearts: Family and Friend's Guide to Breast Cancer Support" serves as a trusted companion for those seeking to provide unwavering support to their loved ones facing breast cancer. Whether you are a family member, friend, or caregiver, this book offers valuable insights, practical strategies, and empathetic guidance to help you navigate the challenges of the breast cancer journey together.

Chapter 1: The Breast Cancer Journey

Overview of Breast Cancer: Types, Stages, and Treatments

Breast cancer is a complicated and complex illness that influences a huge number of people around the world. This chapter provides an essential overview of breast cancer, including its various types, stages, and available treatments. Understanding these fundamental aspects is crucial for both patients and their support network to make informed decisions and offer effective assistance.

Types of Breast Cancer:

Ductal Carcinoma In Situ (DCIS): This early-stage cancer originates in the milk ducts and is confined within them. It is considered non-invasive.

Invasive Ductal Carcinoma (IDC): The most widely recognized kind of breast cancer, IDC begins in the milk conduits and afterward attacks encompassing tissues.

Invasive Lobular Carcinoma (ILC): This cancer begins in the milk-producing glands and can spread to nearby tissues.

HER2-Positive Breast Cancer: Some breast cancers produce too much of a protein called HER2, which can promote the growth of cancer cells.

Triple-Negative Breast Cancer: This type lacks receptors for estrogen, progesterone, and HER2, making it harder to treat.

Stages of Breast Cancer:

Breast cancer is categorized into stages based on the size of the tumor, lymph node involvement, and whether it has spread to other parts of the body.

Stage 0: Non-invasive cancers, like DCIS, are confined within the ducts or lobules.

Stage I and II: These stages involve invasive cancers that have spread to nearby tissues or lymph nodes.

Stage III: Cancer is locally advanced and may have spread to multiple lymph nodes or tissues nearby.

Stage IV: Advanced metastatic cancer, where cancer has spread to distant organs like the lungs, liver, or bones.

Treatments for Breast Cancer:

Surgery: Lumpectomy (removal of the tumor) or mastectomy (removal of the breast) are common surgical options.

Radiation Therapy: High-energy rays target and kill cancer cells, often after surgery.

Chemotherapy: Drugs are used to kill or slow the growth of cancer cells throughout the body.

Hormone Therapy: If the cancer is hormone-receptor-positive, drugs are used to block the effects of hormones that fuel cancer growth.

Targeted Therapy: Drugs like Herceptin target specific proteins to inhibit cancer growth.

Immunotherapy: Boosting the body's immune system to fight cancer cells.

Understanding the different types, stages, and treatment options for breast cancer provides a foundation for effective support. By being informed, caregivers and loved ones can better assist patients in their treatment decisions and recovery process. This knowledge empowers everyone involved to actively participate in the journey toward overcoming breast cancer's challenges.

Emotional Rollercoaster: Dealing with Diagnosis and Initial Reactions

The moment of receiving a breast cancer diagnosis is often a life-altering event that triggers a wide range of intense emotions. This chapter explores the emotional rollercoaster that patients face upon diagnosis and offers insights into how both patients and their support network can navigate this challenging phase with empathy and understanding.

Shock and Disbelief: The initial reaction to a breast cancer diagnosis is often shock and disbelief. The unexpected acknowledgment of confronting a dangerous disease can overpower. Patients may struggle to process the information and find it hard to believe that such a diagnosis could apply to them.

Fear and Anxiety: Fear of the unknown and the uncertainty of the future can lead to heightened anxiety. Thoughts about treatment, potential side effects, and how life will change can dominate a patient's mind. The fear of the impact on loved ones and day-to-day responsibilities can also intensify these emotions.

Sadness and Grief: The news of a breast cancer diagnosis can trigger feelings of profound sadness and grief. Patients mourn the loss of their previous sense of health and well-being, as well as the disruption to their life plans.

Anger and Frustration: Some individuals experience anger, questioning why they are facing such a challenging situation. Feelings of frustration can arise from the perception of injustice or an inability to control what is happening.

Denial and Avoidance: Coping mechanisms such as denial or avoidance may manifest as attempts to distance oneself from the diagnosis. Patients might downplay the severity of the situation or avoid discussing it altogether.

Empathy and Support: For caregivers and loved ones, understanding these initial reactions is crucial. Offering a compassionate and non-judgmental presence can help patients process their emotions. Active listening, validation of feelings, and reassurance that their emotions are valid can provide comfort.

Encouraging Open Dialogue: Creating a safe space for patients to express their emotions is essential. Encouraging open dialogue allows patients to share their fears and concerns, fostering an environment of trust and understanding.

Balancing Positivity: While acknowledging the intense emotions, finding moments of positivity can be helpful. Encouraging patients to focus on their strengths, celebrate small victories, and find sources of joy can help balance the emotional scale.

Seeking Professional Help: It's important to recognize when emotional distress becomes overwhelming. Encourage patients to seek professional support, such as therapists or counselors, to help them healthily process their emotions.

In conclusion, the period following a breast cancer diagnosis is marked by a rollercoaster of emotions. Patients need patience, empathy, and understanding from their support network as they navigate this tumultuous phase. By offering genuine emotional support and being a source of strength, caregivers and loved ones can help patients gradually find their footing and begin to cope with the challenges that lie ahead.

Chapter 2: Navigating Supportive Roles

The Role of Family and Friends in the Journey

The journey through breast cancer is not one that individuals face alone; it's a path that is walked with the support, love, and care of family and friends. This chapter explores the vital role that family members and friends play in the breast cancer journey, highlighting the importance of their presence, understanding, and unwavering support.

Pillars of Strength: Family and friends often serve as pillars of strength for individuals facing breast cancer. Their presence provides a source of comfort and reassurance during challenging times.

Emotional Support: One of the most significant roles of family and friends is to provide emotional support. Listening without judgment, offering a shoulder to cry on, and providing a safe space for expressing fears and concerns all contribute to the patient's emotional well-being.

Advocacy and Communication: Loved ones can act as advocates on behalf of the patient, ensuring that medical concerns and questions are addressed. They can accompany the patient to medical appointments, help clarify information, and ensure that the patient's voice is heard.

Providing Practical Assistance: Family and friends can help alleviate the daily burdens that come with a breast cancer diagnosis. Assisting with household chores, cooking meals, and running errands can provide much-needed relief for patients who might be dealing with fatigue or side effects from treatment.

Maintaining Normalcy: Amidst the upheaval caused by a breast cancer diagnosis, loved ones can help maintain a sense of normalcy. Engaging in activities that the patient enjoys and spending quality time together can provide a sense of continuity and joy.

Being Informed and Empathetic: Family and friends who take the time to educate themselves about breast cancer can better understand the patient's experience. This knowledge fosters empathy and enables them to provide relevant and meaningful support.

Navigating Difficult Conversations: Difficult conversations about treatment options, prognosis, and fears are an integral part of the journey. Family and friends can help patients navigate these conversations, offering a supportive presence and helping them process complex information.

Offering Hope and Positivity: Loved ones can be a source of hope and positivity. By focusing on the patient's strengths, achievements, and milestones, they can help uplift the patient's spirits and reinforce their resilience.

Self-Care for Caregivers: Family and friends need to remember that caregiving can take a toll on their well-being. Prioritizing self-care and seeking support from their network can ensure that they can provide effective support.

Celebrating Milestones: Celebrating both small and significant milestones in the patient's journey showcases the power of support. These celebrations reinforce the patient's progress and the shared determination to overcome challenges.

In conclusion, the role of family and friends in the breast cancer journey is invaluable. Their support, love, and understanding can significantly impact the patient's emotional well-being and overall experience. By standing by their side with empathy, compassion, and strength, family members and friends play an essential role in uplifting spirits and healing hearts throughout the breast cancer journey.

Communicating Effectively: Being Present and Listening

Effective communication is a cornerstone of providing support to individuals facing breast cancer. This chapter delves into the art of communicating with empathy, focusing on being present, actively listening, and creating a space where patients can express their thoughts and feelings openly.

The Power of Presence:

Being physically and emotionally present communicates care and support. Your presence alone can offer comfort, even when words are hard to find.

Active Listening:

Listen Without Interruption: When patients share their thoughts, allow them to speak without interruption. This shows that you value what they're saying.

Show Genuine Interest: Ask open-ended questions that encourage them to share more about their feelings and experiences. Your genuine interest makes them feel heard and understood.

Reflect: Occasionally paraphrase or reflect on what they've said. This demonstrates that you're actively engaged in the conversation and seeking to understand.

Create a Safe Space:

Non-Judgmental Environment: Create an environment where patients feel safe sharing their emotions, fears, and concerns without fearing judgment.

Avoid Offering Solutions Immediately: Sometimes, patients just need a space to vent. Instead of jumping to solutions, listen first and ask if they'd like advice or assistance.

Be Mindful of Nonverbal Communication:

Eye Contact: Maintain appropriate eye contact to show your attentiveness and sincerity.

Body Language: Your body language should reflect your engagement. Avoid crossing your arms or looking distracted.

Empathetic Responses:

Acknowledge Emotions: Validating their emotions with statements like "I can imagine how challenging that must be" lets them know you understand.

Offer Reassurance: Providing reassurance that they're not alone and you're there to support them can be immensely comforting.

Use Open and Honest Communication:

Be Transparent: If you're unsure how to respond or support, it's okay to say so. Honesty shows that you're genuine and willing to learn.

Express Your Feelings: Share your own emotions, but avoid making the conversation about yourself. A basic "I'm hanging around for you" can go quite far.

Respect Silence and Space:
Not every moment requires conversation. Sometimes, silence is a powerful way to show your support. Allow patients the space they need without pressuring them to speak.

Follow Their Lead:
Patients may have varying comfort levels when it comes to discussing their diagnosis. Respect their boundaries and follow their lead in terms of how much they're willing to share.

In conclusion, effective communication is a foundation of support during the breast cancer journey. By being present, actively listening, and creating a safe and empathetic space, you provide patients with the emotional support they need to navigate this challenging time. Your willingness to communicate openly and sincerely can make a significant impact on their well-being and their ability to cope with the challenges ahead.

Chapter 3: Providing Practical Help

Assisting with Daily Activities: Cooking, Cleaning, and More

When a loved one is facing breast cancer, everyday tasks can become overwhelming due to treatment side effects and fatigue. This chapter explores the importance of providing practical assistance with daily activities and offers insights into how caregivers and friends can help alleviate the burdens of cooking, cleaning, and other essential tasks.

Understanding the Impact of Treatment:

Fatigue: Treatment often leads to extreme fatigue, making even simple tasks feel exhausting.

Side Effects: Patients may experience nausea, weakness, and pain, affecting their ability to perform daily activities.

Offering Assistance:

Meal Preparation: Cooking nutritious meals can be challenging. Preparing or delivering ready-to-eat meals helps ensure the patient receives proper nutrition.

Grocery Shopping: Help with grocery shopping or even order groceries online for their convenience.

Cleaning and Chores: Assist with household cleaning, laundry, and other chores to keep their living space comfortable and stress-free.

Child and Pet Care: Taking care of children and pets can be demanding. Offering to babysit or walk pets provides much-needed relief.

Creating a Support Schedule:

Coordinate with Others: Communicate with family and friends to create a support schedule that ensures the patient receives consistent help without overwhelming any one individual.

Rotating Tasks: Assign different tasks to different people to share the load and prevent burnout.

Adapt to Their Preferences:

Respect Their Independence: While offering assistance, be sensitive to their desire for independence. Ask if they would like help before stepping in.

Flexible Approach: Be adaptable. Patients' needs may change daily, so be ready to adjust your assistance accordingly.

Offer Emotional Support While Assisting

Quality Time: Engaging in conversations while assisting with tasks can provide emotional support and create a sense of normalcy.

Positive Atmosphere: Creating a cheerful environment while cooking, cleaning, or helping can uplift their spirits.

Empower Their Choices:

Meal Preferences: When preparing meals, respect their dietary preferences and restrictions.

Cleaning Style: If helping with cleaning, ask how they prefer their living space organized and cleaned.

Maintain Their Dignity:

Privacy and Boundaries: Respect their privacy by asking before entering certain spaces or assisting with personal tasks.

Encourage Independence: Support their efforts to do tasks independently when they feel up to it.

In conclusion, offering assistance with daily activities is a practical and impactful way to support a loved one facing breast cancer. By alleviating the stress of cooking, cleaning, and other tasks, you contribute to their overall well-being and allow them to focus on their recovery. Your thoughtfulness, flexibility, and empathy demonstrate your commitment to walking beside them on this challenging journey.

Transportation and Medical Appointments: A Helping Hand

Navigating medical appointments and transportation can be a significant challenge for individuals facing breast cancer. This chapter delves into the importance of providing assistance with transportation and attending medical appointments, offering insights into how family and friends can play a vital role in ensuring that patients receive the care they need.

The Impact of Treatment on Mobility:

Physical Effects: Treatment side effects such as fatigue, nausea, and weakness can make driving and using public transportation difficult.

Precautions: Some treatments might require patients to refrain from driving due to drowsiness or dizziness.

The Role of Caregivers and Loved Ones:

Reliable Transportation: Offering rides to medical appointments ensures that patients can access treatment without stress.

Emotional Support: Being there for medical appointments provides emotional support during what can be anxiety-inducing visits.

Practical Assistance:

Navigating the Healthcare System: Offer help with scheduling appointments, understanding directions, and filling out paperwork.

Waiting Room Support: Accompany patients to appointments and be a comforting presence while they wait.

Creating a Supportive Environment:

Preparation: Discuss the upcoming appointment with the patient to ensure they have all necessary documents and questions ready.

Stay Organized: Keep track of appointment dates, times, and locations to ensure punctuality.

Safety and Comfort:

Accommodate Special Needs: If patients have mobility challenges, ensure that the vehicle is accessible or that appropriate assistance is available.

Bring Comfort Items: Carry snacks, water, and any comfort items they might need during appointments.

Open Communication:

Discuss Their Preferences: Check if they would like company during appointments or if they prefer some alone time.

Understand Their Concerns: Be prepared to listen and offer reassurance if they're nervous about the appointment.

Maintain Privacy and Confidentiality:

Respect Boundaries: While being supportive, respect their privacy during medical visits.

Confidentiality: Refrain from sharing any personal or medical information without their consent.

Offering Post-Appointment Assistance:

Recovery Period: Some treatments might leave patients feeling tired or unwell after appointments. Offering a ride home and helping with immediate needs can be incredibly helpful.

Following Doctor's Orders: Remind them to follow post-appointment instructions and take prescribed medications.

In conclusion, providing transportation and attending medical appointments with loved ones facing breast cancer is a crucial way to offer support. By being a reliable and comforting presence, you ensure that patients can focus on their care and treatment without worrying about logistical challenges. Your willingness to navigate the healthcare system and create a supportive environment reflects your commitment to their well-being during this challenging journey.

Chapter 4: Emotional Support

Being an Empathetic Presence: Expressing Care and Empathy

In the journey through breast cancer, being an empathetic presence is a powerful way to provide meaningful support. This chapter delves into the significance of expressing care and empathy, offering insights into how family and friends can genuinely connect with patients, fostering an atmosphere of understanding and emotional comfort.

The Impact of Empathy:

Emotional Resonance: Expressing empathy allows you to connect emotionally with the patient, creating a sense of shared understanding.

Validation: Feeling heard and understood validates the patient's emotions and experiences, reducing feelings of isolation.

Ways to Be an Empathetic Presence:

Active Listening: Pay full attention when they speak, without interrupting or formulating responses. This shows that you esteem their considerations and sentiments.

Nonverbal Cues: Maintain eye contact, nod, and use appropriate facial expressions to show you're engaged in the conversation.

Mirroring Emotions: Reflect their emotions to them. If they express sadness, you might say, "It sounds like you're feeling really sad right now."

Offering Reassurance: Use phrases like "I'm here for you" and "You're not alone" to reassure them that you're by their side.

Empathy in Action:

Ask Open-Ended Questions: Encourage them to share their thoughts and feelings with questions like "How are you feeling today?" or "What's been on your mind?"

Practice Emotional Validation: Instead of minimizing their emotions, validate their feelings by saying, "It's completely normal to feel that way."

Use Their Language: If they use certain words to describe their emotions, incorporate those words into your responses. This shows you're truly listening.

Avoid Comparison or Offering Solutions:

Steer Clear of Comparisons: Avoid statements like "I know how you feel," as each person's experience is unique.

Listen Without Fixing: While your intention may be to help, sometimes they just need someone to listen and empathize, without offering solutions.

Share Your Own Emotions, When Appropriate:

Common Experiences: If you've faced similar challenges, sharing your emotions can help them feel less alone.

Keep the Focus on Them: While sharing your experiences can be comforting, ensure that the conversation remains centered on their needs.

Respecting Their Pace:

Allow Silence: Sometimes, they might need a moment to gather their thoughts. Allow space for silence without feeling compelled to fill it.

Be Patient: If they're not ready to talk about certain topics, respect their pace and give them time.

In conclusion, being an empathetic presence involves more than just offering words of comfort—it's about creating a connection that makes patients feel heard, understood, and cared for. By practicing active listening, validating emotions, and showing genuine concern, you contribute to their emotional well-being and provide a safe space for them to share their feelings. Your empathetic presence is a valuable source of strength and support throughout the breast cancer journey.

Managing Tough Conversations and Providing Comfort

In the face of breast cancer, having difficult conversations becomes an inevitable part of the journey. This chapter explores the importance of managing these conversations with sensitivity and compassion, as well as offering comfort to patients in times of emotional distress.

The Need for Tough Conversations:

Treatment Decisions: Discussions about treatment options, potential side effects, and risks are essential for informed decision-making.

Prognosis: Addressing concerns about prognosis and potential outcomes can be challenging but necessary.

Approaching Tough Conversations:

Choose the Right Setting: Find a quiet, comfortable space where you can talk without distractions.

Ask Permission: Begin by asking if they're ready to talk about a specific topic. This provides them with a feeling of control.

Use Open-Ended Questions: Encourage them to share their thoughts with questions like "What are your concerns about the treatment options?"

Active Listening: Show that you're fully engaged by listening intently and acknowledging their feelings.

Providing Comfort During Tough Conversations:

Reassurance: Remind them that you're there to support them no matter what decisions they make.

Empathy: Use phrases like "I can't fully understand, but I'm here to listen" to express empathy.

Validation: Validate their emotions by saying "It's okay to feel scared" or "Your feelings are completely normal."

Offering Comfort During Emotional Moments:

Create a Safe Space: Let them know that they can express their emotions freely without judgment.

Physical Comfort: Sometimes, a gentle hug or holding their hand can provide immense comfort.

Empathetic Silence: Sometimes, sitting silently and offering a comforting presence is enough.

Remaining Calm and Patient:

Stay Composed: If they become emotional, stay calm and composed. Your steadiness can offer a sense of security.

Patient Listening: Allow them to express themselves fully without rushing to respond.

Knowing When to Seek Professional Help:

Recognize Your Limits: If a conversation becomes overwhelming, it's okay to suggest seeking professional counseling.

Offer Support: Encourage them to seek counseling or therapy if they're struggling to cope.

Follow Up:

Check-In: After tough conversations, follow up to see how they're feeling and if they have any questions.

Offer Resources: Share relevant books, websites, or support groups that can provide additional information or assistance.

In conclusion, managing tough conversations and providing comfort are essential skills in supporting individuals facing breast cancer. By approaching these discussions with sensitivity, empathy, and patience, you create a safe space for them to share their fears, concerns, and hopes. Your willingness to be there during difficult moments and your ability to offer solace make a significant impact on their emotional well-being and their ability to cope with the challenges ahead.

Chapter 5: Creating a Supportive Environment

Maintaining Positivity and Hope: Fostering a Supportive Atmosphere

Positivity and hope are powerful allies in the breast cancer journey, providing strength and resilience. This chapter explores the significance of maintaining a positive outlook and creating a supportive atmosphere, offering insights into how family and friends can contribute to fostering a sense of hope and optimism.

The Impact of Positivity and Hope:

Psychological Well-being: A positive attitude can enhance psychological well-being and reduce stress.

Resilience: Maintaining hope fosters resilience, allowing individuals to better navigate challenges.

Ways to Foster Positivity and Hope:

Celebrate Achievements: Acknowledge even small milestones, like completing a treatment or a successful medical check-up.

Focus on Strengths: Highlight their strengths, both physical and emotional, to boost their confidence.

Share Success Stories: Share stories of breast cancer survivors who have overcome challenges to inspire hope.

Creating a Supportive Atmosphere:

Embrace Moments of Joy: Incorporate laughter and joyful activities into their routine.

Stay Engaged: Engage in conversations that revolve around positive experiences, hobbies, or plans.

Offering Encouragement and Affirmations:

Daily Affirmations: Help them develop a list of positive affirmations to recite daily.

Words of Encouragement: Share uplifting quotes or messages that remind them of their inner strength.

Sharing Positive News and Stories:

Highlight Progress: If they've made progress in their treatment or recovery, celebrate and share the news.

Inspirational Content: Share articles, videos, or books that focus on healing resilience, and positive outcomes.

Being a Source of Light:

Acts of Kindness: Perform unexpected acts of kindness to brighten their day.

Bringing Joy: Organize activities or outings that bring joy, distraction, and positive experiences.

Maintaining Hope in Tough Times:

Resilience in Adversity: Remind them of their strength to persevere even in difficult moments.

Emphasize Progress: Focus on how far they've come and the potential for brighter days ahead.

Cultivating a Hopeful Mindset:

Visualizations: Encourage them to visualize positive outcomes and a future free from illness.

Mindfulness and Gratitude: Practice mindfulness and gratitude exercises to foster positivity.

In conclusion, maintaining positivity and hope is a collaborative effort that involves both patients and their support network. By creating a supportive atmosphere that focuses on strengths, celebrates achievements, and emphasizes the potential for a brighter future, family and friends play an essential role in cultivating a hopeful mindset. Your efforts to infuse their journey with positivity and hope contribute to their overall well-being and inspire them to face the challenges of breast cancer with strength and determination.

Celebrating Milestones: Joy amid Challenges

In the journey through breast cancer, celebrating milestones takes on a special significance. This chapter delves into the importance of acknowledging and commemorating both small and significant milestones, offering insights into how family and friends can infuse moments of joy and positivity into the midst of challenges.

Why Celebrate Milestones:

Boosting Morale: Recognizing achievements uplifts spirits, fostering a positive outlook.

Building Resilience: Celebrating milestones strengthens the patient's determination to overcome challenges.

Identifying Milestones:

Treatment Progress: Marking milestones like completing a round of treatment or reaching a specific phase can provide a sense of accomplishment.

Anniversaries: Celebrate the anniversary of important events, like the day of diagnosis or the start of treatment, to reflect on progress.

Ways to Celebrate:

Simple Gestures: Arrange a small gathering, send flowers, or give a heartfelt card to mark the occasion.

Create Memory Journals: Encourage them to keep a journal of milestones reached, documenting their journey's highs and lows.

Shared Moments of Joy:

Incorporate Hobbies: Engage in activities they enjoy, like cooking a favorite meal or spending time outdoors.

Quality Time: Spend quality time together, engaging in conversations that bring laughter and positivity.

Planning Future Events:

Bucket List: Help them create a bucket list of things they want to do once they've overcome their challenges.

Dreaming Big: Encourage them to envision future milestones like family gatherings, trips, or special occasions.

Involving the Support Network:

Family and Friends: Invite loved ones to join in the celebrations, making them feel supported and cherished.

Virtual Gatherings: If in-person gatherings aren't feasible, arrange virtual celebrations to connect across distances.

Acknowledge Small Victories:

Daily Triumphs: Recognize the everyday achievements, like completing exercises or managing side effects.

Mindset Shifts: Celebrate mindset shifts, where they're able to view challenges in a more positive light.

Reflecting on Progress:

Progress Journal: Create a journal that documents milestones reached and reflections on the journey.

Gratitude Practice: Encourage them to practice gratitude by listing things they're grateful for on each milestone.

Continuing the Tradition:

Ongoing Celebration: As they move forward, continue to acknowledge new milestones in their journey.

Annual Reflection: Set aside a time each year to reflect on the progress made and the achievements attained.

In conclusion, celebrating milestones offers a chance to find joy and positivity amidst the challenges of breast cancer. Recognizing achievements, fostering a supportive atmosphere, and involving loved ones, family and friends can contribute to moments of happiness and empowerment. Your efforts to celebrate their journey's highs and commemorate their progress remind them that every step forward is a triumph worth celebrating, reinforcing their resilience and determination to overcome breast cancer's obstacles.

Chapter 6: Self-Care for Caregivers

The Importance of Caring for Yourself

While supporting a loved one through breast cancer is crucial, it's equally important to care for yourself. This chapter delves into the significance of self-care, offering insights into how taking care of your physical, emotional, and mental well-being enables you to provide better support to the patient and maintain your health.

The Role of Self-Care:

Sustain Your Well-being: Prioritizing self-care ensures you have the physical and emotional energy needed to provide effective support.

Prevent Burnout: Caring for yourself prevents burnout, allowing you to provide consistent assistance without feeling overwhelmed.

Physical Self-Care:

Healthy Diet: Proper nutrition supports your energy levels and overall well-being.

Regular Exercise: Physical activity boosts mood, reduces stress, and improves your physical health.

Adequate Rest: Getting enough sleep is essential for your mental and physical health.

Emotional Self-Care:

Processing Emotions: Allow yourself to feel your emotions and seek outlets for processing them, such as journaling or talking to a friend.

Setting Boundaries: Clearly define your role and limits to prevent emotional exhaustion.

Practice Self-Compassion: Treat yourself with the same kindness you offer others.

Mental Self-Care:

Mindfulness and Meditation: Engage in mindfulness practices to reduce stress and increase self-awareness.

Engaging Hobbies: Pursuing hobbies you enjoy provides a positive outlet for relaxation.

Limit Media Exposure: While staying informed is important, limit exposure to distressing news or stories.

Seeking Support for Yourself:

Talk to Someone: Confide with a friend, family member, or therapist about your feelings and concerns.

Join Support Groups: Connect with others who are in similar caregiving roles to share experiences and coping strategies.

Guilt and Self-Care:

Release Guilt: Understand that taking care of yourself doesn't diminish your dedication to the patient; it enhances it.

Model Healthy Behavior: By practicing self-care, you set a positive example for the patient to follow.

Balancing Caregiving and Self-Care:

Schedule Self-Care: Set aside regular times for self-care activities and honor them as you would any other commitment.

Delegate When Possible: Enlist the help of other family members or friends to share caregiving responsibilities.

Staying Informed:

Educate Yourself: Learn about breast cancer, its treatments, and how you can best support your loved one.

Setting Realistic Expectations: Understand that your ability to provide support might vary based on your circumstances and limitations.

In conclusion, caring for yourself is not selfish; it's essential. By prioritizing your well-being through physical, emotional, and mental self-care, you ensure that you're better equipped to provide effective support to your loved one facing breast cancer. Remember that taking care of yourself enables you to offer sustained care, empathy, and assistance, creating a healthier and more supportive environment for both you and the patient.

Coping Strategies and Seeking Outside Support

Supporting a loved one through breast cancer can be emotionally demanding. This chapter explores coping strategies and the importance of seeking outside support, providing insights into how caregivers and friends can effectively manage their own emotions and well-being while providing unwavering support.

The Significance of Coping Strategies:

Stress Management: Coping strategies help you manage stress, anxiety, and other challenging emotions.

Sustaining Support: Effective coping ensures you can provide sustained and consistent support to your loved one.

Healthy Coping Strategies:

Deep Breathing and Meditation: Engage in deep breathing exercises or meditation to reduce stress and promote relaxation.

Exercise: Physical activity releases endorphins, boosting your mood and overall well-being.

Journaling: Write down your thoughts and emotions as a way to process them.

Time Management: Create a structured routine that balances caregiving and self-care activities.

Art and Creativity: Engage in artistic pursuits as an outlet for emotional expression.

Recognizing Unhealthy Coping Mechanisms:

Avoiding Emotions: Suppressing emotions can lead to emotional exhaustion.

Overworking: Excessive caregiving without self-care can lead to burnout.

Seeking Outside Support:

Therapy and Counseling: Speak to a therapist or counselor about your feelings, fears, and challenges.

Support Groups: Join support groups for caregivers to connect with others who understand your experiences.

Setting Boundaries and Asking for Help:

Define Boundaries: Communicate your limits to prevent emotional and physical exhaustion.

Delegate Responsibilities: Enlist the help of family, friends, or hired assistance to share caregiving tasks.

Recognizing Signs of Burnout:

Emotional Exhaustion: Feeling emotionally drained or detached from the situation.

Physical Symptoms: Experiencing fatigue, headaches, or changes in sleep patterns.

The Importance of Self-Compassion:

Treat Yourself Kindly: Avoid self-criticism and practice self-compassion.

Prioritize Self-Care: Remember that taking care of yourself is not selfish; it's necessary for effective caregiving.

Balancing Your Needs and Responsibilities:

Time for Self-Care: Dedicate regular time to engage in self-care activities without guilt.

Open Communication: Discuss your emotional well-being with your loved one, so they understand your needs too.

Understanding Your Limits:

You're Human: Accept that you have limitations and can't always provide all the answers or solutions.

Support for Yourself: Seek professional help if you find yourself struggling with your mental health.

In conclusion, coping strategies and seeking outside support are essential components of effectively providing care for a loved one with breast cancer. By adopting healthy coping mechanisms, recognizing the signs of burnout, and seeking assistance when needed, you ensure that you're able to maintain your well-being while offering meaningful and sustained support. Remember that taking care of yourself not only benefits you but also enhances your ability to be a pillar of strength for your loved one throughout their breast cancer journey.

Chapter 7: Navigating Treatment and Recovery

Chemotherapy, Radiation, and Surgery: What to Expect

Understanding the different treatment options for breast cancer is crucial in providing support to your loved one. This chapter provides insights into what to expect during chemotherapy, radiation therapy, and surgery, helping you offer informed and empathetic support throughout your treatment journey.

Chemotherapy:

Purpose: Chemotherapy uses powerful drugs to destroy cancer cells or slow their growth.

Treatment Schedule: It's typically given in cycles, with periods of rest in between.

Side Effects: Common side effects include fatigue, nausea, hair loss, and changes in appetite.

Supportive Care: Offer assistance with transportation to and from appointments, meal preparation, and emotional support during challenging side effects.

Radiation Therapy:

Purpose: Radiation therapy uses high-energy rays to target and destroy cancer cells.

Treatment Schedule: Usually administered daily over a set period, often for a few weeks.

Side Effects: Skin irritation, fatigue, and localized discomfort are common side effects.

Supportive Care: Provide comfort during periods of discomfort, assist with transportation, and help with any daily activities that may become difficult.

Surgery:

Purpose: Surgery aims to remove the tumor and surrounding tissue from the breast.

Types of Surgery: Lumpectomy (removal of tumor and some tissue) or mastectomy (removal of the entire breast) are common options.

Recovery: Recovery varies based on the type of surgery. Support during the mending system is urgent.

Emotional Impact: Surgery can have emotional implications due to changes in body image. Offer empathy and understanding.

Support Strategies:

Accompany to Appointments: Offer to accompany your loved one to medical appointments for emotional support and to help them remember information.

Ask about Treatment Plan: Understand their treatment plan so you can anticipate their needs during different phases.

Manage Medications: Help them keep track of medications, appointments, and any instructions from healthcare providers.

Create a Comfortable Environment: Ensure their home environment is conducive to rest and recovery, especially after surgery.

Emotional Support: Be a listening ear, offering encouragement and understanding during challenging times.

Handling Emotions:

Acknowledge Their Feelings: Recognize their emotions and reassure them that their feelings are valid.

Provide a Safe Space: Encourage them to share their concerns without judgment.

Educate Yourself:

Learn About Treatments: Understanding the treatments will enable you to answer questions and provide reassurance.

Know the Side Effects: Being aware of potential side effects allows you to offer appropriate support and assistance.

In conclusion, supporting a loved one through chemotherapy, radiation therapy, and surgery involves being informed, empathetic, and attentive to their needs. By understanding the treatment process, being a pillar of emotional support, and assisting with practical aspects of their journey, you contribute to their overall well-being and help alleviate some of the challenges they may face during breast cancer treatment.

Providing Help During Treatment and Rehabilitation

Supporting your loved one during breast cancer treatment and rehabilitation is a vital aspect of their journey. This chapter offers insights into how you can effectively provide assistance, comfort, and encouragement during this phase, ensuring that they receive the care they need to navigate their treatment and recovery.

Accompanying to Appointments:

Emotional Support: Offer to accompany them to medical appointments, providing comfort and an extra pair of ears to understand treatment plans.

Note-Taking: Take notes during appointments to help them remember important information and instructions.

Medication Management:

Organize Medications: Help them keep track of medications and adhere to prescribed schedules.

Address Side Effects: Assist in managing side effects by ensuring they take medications as directed.

Managing Symptoms and Side Effects:

Nutritional Support: Prepare meals that align with their dietary needs and preferences.

Hydration: Encourage regular hydration, which is important during treatment.

Comfort Measures: Provide items that alleviate side effects, such as skin creams for radiation-related irritation.

Emotional and Mental Well-being:

Engage in Uplifting Activities: Participate in activities they enjoy to boost their mood.

Provide Distraction: Engage them in conversations or activities that take their mind off treatment-related stress.

Assisting with Rehabilitation:

Physical Therapy Support: Accompany them with physical therapy sessions and help with exercises at home.

Mobility Assistance: Offer help with tasks that might be physically challenging during recovery.

Create a Comfortable Recovery Space:

Prepare the Home: Ensure their living space is conducive to rest and recovery after treatments.

Provide Entertainment: Offer books, movies, or hobbies to keep them occupied during downtime.

Encouragement and Celebration:

Acknowledge Milestones: Celebrate achievements and treatment milestones to boost their morale.

Emphasize Progress: Remind them of the progress they've made and the strength they've shown.

Offering Social Support:

Arrange Social Interactions: Coordinate visits or virtual interactions with friends and family to keep their spirits up.

Listening Ear: Be available to listen to their feelings and concerns without judgment.

Balancing Independence and Assistance:

Respect Independence: Encourage them to do tasks on their own when they're up to it.

Offer Assistance: Be ready to step in when they need help without making them feel dependent.

Educate Yourself and Communicate Openly:

Stay Informed: Learn about the different phases of treatment and recovery to offer informed support.

Ask for Preferences: Understand their needs and preferences for assistance, respecting their wishes.

In conclusion, providing help during breast cancer treatment and rehabilitation involves a combination of practical assistance, emotional support, and open communication. By being attentive to their needs, helping manage side effects, and creating a supportive environment, you play a crucial role in their recovery journey. Your presence, care, and willingness to adapt to their changing needs contribute significantly to their well-being and overall sense of comfort.

Chapter 8: Long-Term Support

Life After Treatment: Emotional and Physical Adjustments

The completion of breast cancer treatment marks a significant milestone, but it also brings about new challenges as your loved one enters the phase of life after treatment. This chapter explores the emotional and physical adjustments that may arise during this period and provides insights on how you can continue to offer meaningful support as they transition to this new chapter.

Emotional Adjustments:

Mixed Emotions: It's normal to experience a mix of relief, happiness, and anxiety about the future after treatment ends.

Fear of Recurrence: This fear is common. Offer reassurance and remind them to focus on regular follow-up appointments.

Body Image Concerns: Breast cancer treatments may impact physical appearance. Empower them to embrace their bodies and offer emotional support during this adjustment.

Dealing with Change: Acknowledge the changes they've gone through, and encourage open conversations about their feelings.

Physical Adjustments:

Managing Side Effects: Some side effects may persist post-treatment. Help them cope with these effects and ensure they follow up with healthcare providers.

Fatigue: Fatigue can linger. Encourage a balanced routine that includes rest and physical activity.

Physical Recovery: If surgery was involved, they may need time to recover physically. Offer help with day-to-day assignments if necessary.

Lifestyle Changes: Encourage healthy habits, such as a balanced diet, regular exercise, and stress reduction.

Supporting a Positive Outlook:

Encourage Gratitude: Help them focus on the positive aspects of life and celebrate each day.

Future Plans: Assist in planning enjoyable activities, trips, or new hobbies to create a sense of anticipation.

Counseling and Support Groups:

Consider Professional Help: Encourage them to explore therapy or counseling if they struggle with emotional adjustments.

Support Groups: Connect them with breast cancer survivor support groups for shared experiences and emotional support.

Maintaining a Healthy Lifestyle

Encourage Regular Check-ups: Reinforce the importance of follow-up appointments and screenings.

Promote Self-Care: Remind them to continue practicing self-care and managing stress.

Celebrating Survivorship:1

Acknowledge Strength: Remind them of their resilience and strength throughout the journey.

Share Success Stories: Share stories of breast cancer survivors who have thrived post-treatment.

Listening and Understanding

Be Patient: Allow them to express their emotions and concerns without judgment.

Be Available: Continue to be a listening ear, offering your support whenever they need it.

Balancing Independence and Assistance

Encourage Independence: Support their desire to regain independence while being ready to assist when necessary.

Be Adaptable: Recognize that their needs may continue to change, and be willing to adapt your support accordingly.

In conclusion, life after breast cancer treatment brings about a period of emotional and physical adjustments. By understanding these challenges, offering empathy, and helping them maintain a positive outlook, you provide invaluable support as they navigate this new phase of their journey. Your unwavering presence, compassion, and willingness to adapt to their needs contribute to their overall well-being and resilience in embracing life beyond treatment.

Continuing the Journey: Celebrating Survival and Moving Forward

Reaching the point of survival after breast cancer treatment is a remarkable accomplishment, and this phase marks a transition into a new chapter filled with hope and possibilities. This chapter explores the significance of celebrating this achievement and how you can support your loved one in moving forward with optimism, empowerment, and a renewed focus on living life to the fullest.

Celebrating Survival

Acknowledge Strength: Celebrate the courage, resilience, and determination they've demonstrated throughout the breast cancer journey.

Survivorship Milestones: Mark survivorship milestones with meaningful gestures or events that commemorate their triumph over breast cancer.

Embracing Positivity

Reinforce Positivity: Encourage them to embrace a positive outlook on life after surviving breast cancer.

Optimism for the Future: Discuss plans, goals, and dreams to channel their energy towards what lies ahead.

Empowerment and Self-Discovery

Explore New Interests: Encourage them to try new activities or revisit old hobbies, promoting self-discovery.

Focus on Well-being: Assist in maintaining healthy habits, practicing mindfulness, and managing stress.

Supporting Physical Recovery

Physical Activity: Encourage regular exercise to regain strength and enhance overall well-being.

Healthy Lifestyle: Promote a balanced diet, regular check-ups, and adherence to any post-treatment recommendations.

Embracing Body Image

Boosting Confidence: Remind them that their strength and beauty shine through regardless of any physical changes.

Empowerment: Help them focus on what their body has achieved and endured, fostering self-appreciation.

Continuing Relationships

Reconnecting: Encourage them to reconnect with friends and loved ones, rebuilding social connections.

Maintaining Support: Remind them that your support is ongoing, and you're there to celebrate their victories and be a source of comfort whenever needed.

Seeking Professional Support

Counseling: If needed, consider seeking counseling to address any lingering emotional challenges.

Support Groups: Continue engaging with breast cancer survivor support groups for ongoing shared experiences and emotional support.

Future Plans and Aspirations

Setting Goals: Help them set new goals, whether it's a career move, travel, or personal growth.

Dream Big: Encourage them to dream big, embracing the endless possibilities that lie ahead.

Living Each Day Fully

Carpe Diem: Remind them of the importance of seizing the moment and cherishing it every day.

Gratitude: Practice gratitude for the gift of survival and encourage them to appreciate the beauty in life.

In conclusion, celebrating survival after breast cancer treatment is a joyous occasion that should be embraced with enthusiasm and positivity. By offering ongoing support, promoting self-discovery, and helping them focus on the future, you contribute to their continued growth, happiness, and empowerment. Your dedication to their well-being and your shared excitement for the journey ahead is a wonderful gift, helping them embrace life after breast cancer with renewed vigor and gratitude.

Chapter 9: Stories of Strength and Resilience

Personal Accounts from Breast Cancer Survivors and Caregivers

The voices of breast cancer survivors and caregivers offer profound insights into the journey, revealing the strength, resilience, and enduring human spirit that shines even in the face of adversity. In this collection of personal accounts, you'll find stories of courage, hope, and the power of love that provide valuable perspectives for anyone touched by breast cancer.

A Journey of Courage and Resilience

Survivor's Story: Share the inspiring tale of a breast cancer survivor who faced the diagnosis with unwavering courage, navigated the challenges of treatment and emerged with a renewed appreciation for life.

Caregiver's Perspective: Hear from a caregiver who stood by their loved one's side, offering unwavering support, understanding, and comfort during the toughest moments of the journey.

Finding Strength in Unity

Survivor's Triumph: Learn how one survivor's determination, the support of loved ones, and the connection with fellow survivors in support groups created a sense of unity and strength that propelled them forward.

Shared Resilience: Explore a caregiver's perspective on the enduring impact of connecting with other caregivers, sharing experiences, and lifting each other during the challenges of caregiving.

Love, Empathy, and the Journey Forward

Survivor's Reflections: Gain insights into the emotional rollercoaster of a survivor's journey – the fears, the hopes, the moments of vulnerability, and the deep sense of gratitude for the love and support received.

Caregiver's Lessons: Hear from a caregiver about the transformative power of compassion, the importance of self-care, and the enduring connection they've established with their loved one through the trials and triumphs of breast cancer.

Strength in Every Step

Survivor's Triumph Over Challenges: Discover how a survivor faced unexpected obstacles during treatment, yet managed to find strength in the support of caregivers and the unwavering belief in their ability to overcome.

Caregiver's Dedication: Explore a caregiver's commitment to being a steadfast presence, celebrating milestones, and supporting their loved one in reclaiming their life beyond breast cancer.

In these personal accounts, you'll find stories of resilience, love, and the unbreakable bonds forged through the breast cancer journey. These narratives serve as a testament to the human spirit's ability to shine brightly, even in the face of the most challenging circumstances. May these stories inspire you to continue providing the compassionate support that makes such a meaningful difference in the lives of survivors and caregivers.

Chapter 10: Resources and Further Assistance

Support Groups, Online Communities, and Professional Help

In the journey through breast cancer, a strong support system can make all the difference. This chapter highlights the significance of support groups, online communities, and professional help in providing emotional, informational, and practical assistance for individuals and their caregivers, helping them navigate the challenges that arise during this difficult time.

Support Groups

Shared Experiences: Support groups bring together individuals facing similar situations, providing a safe space to share experiences, fears, and triumphs.

Emotional Comfort: Connecting with others who understand their journey can reduce feelings of isolation and offer emotional comfort.

Practical Advice: Members often exchange practical tips and advice on coping with treatment, side effects, and life after cancer.

Personal Growth: Support groups empower individuals to grow emotionally, helping them regain a sense of control and empowerment.

Online Communities

24/7 Access: Online platforms offer continuous support, allowing individuals to connect and share at any time.

Anonymity: Some may find it more comfortable to discuss personal concerns and feelings anonymously in online communities.

Diverse Perspectives: Online communities can provide a wide range of perspectives, allowing individuals to learn from various experiences.

Information Sharing: These communities often share valuable information about the latest treatments, research, and resources.

Professional Help

Therapists and Counselors: Mental health professionals can offer a safe space to process emotions, manage anxiety, and address the psychological impact of breast cancer.

Psychiatrists: When needed, psychiatrists can provide medication management to address mood disorders or severe anxiety.

Social Workers: Social workers can assist with practical concerns, such as navigating healthcare systems, financial challenges, and accessing community resources.

Nutritionists: Nutritional guidance is essential for maintaining health during and after treatment, and nutritionists can offer personalized advice.

When to Seek Professional Help

Overwhelming Emotions: If feelings of anxiety, depression, or distress become overwhelming, professional help is beneficial.

Crisis Situations: In cases of crisis, such as severe emotional distress or suicidal thoughts, immediate professional intervention is necessary.

Complex Issues: When facing complex issues like long-term emotional struggles or challenging family dynamics, professional guidance can be invaluable.

Balancing Different Support Channels

Complementary Support: Support groups, online communities, and professional help can complement each other, offering a well-rounded support system.

Respecting Preferences: Recognize that different individuals may prefer different types of support. Respect their choices and offer assistance accordingly.

In conclusion, support groups, online communities, and professional help play crucial roles in the breast cancer journey. By encouraging access to these resources, you empower individuals and caregivers to navigate challenges, find understanding, and discover the tools necessary to cope with the emotional and practical aspects of breast cancer. Your support in connecting them with these resources demonstrates your commitment to their well-being and ensures they have the assistance they need on this challenging but manageable path.

Additional Reading and References

Expanding your knowledge on breast cancer, caregiving, and survivorship can be incredibly valuable as you continue to support your loved one and navigate the complexities of this journey. This section provides recommendations for additional reading and references that offer comprehensive information, insights, and inspiration.

Books

The Breast Cancer Survival Manual: A Step-By-Step Guide for the Woman With Newly Diagnosed Breast Cancer" by John Link, MD, and James Waisman, MD.

Chicken Soup for the Breast Cancer Survivor's Spirit: Stories to Move, Backing, and Mend" by Jack Canfield, Imprint Victor Hansen, and Mary Olsen Kelly.

Radical Remission: Surviving Cancer Against All Odds" by Kelly A. Turner, Ph.D.

The Cancer-Fighting Kitchen: Nourishing, Big-Flavor Recipes for Cancer Treatment and Recovery" by Rebecca Katz.

Online Resources

American Cancer Society (cancer.org): Comprehensive information on breast cancer, treatment options, coping strategies, and survivorship.

BreastCancer.org: A trusted online resource offering a wealth of information on breast cancer, treatments, clinical trials, and supportive community forums.

National Breast Cancer Foundation (national breastcancer.org): Provides educational resources, early detection tools, and support services.

American Society of Clinical Oncology (cancer.net): Information on cancer treatments, side effects, survivorship, and the latest advancements in oncology.

Support Groups and Forums

Local Support Groups: Check with local hospitals or cancer centers for in-person support groups.

Inspire (inspire.com): An online platform with numerous breast cancer-related support communities where individuals can connect and share experiences.

Breast Cancer Now Forum (forum.breast cancer now.org): A UK-based platform that offers discussion forums for those affected by breast cancer.

Professional Organizations:

Oncology Nurses Society (ONS): Offers resources on cancer care, patient education, and treatment updates.

Relationship of Oncology Social Work (AOSW): Gives data on psychosocial care, backing, and assets for people with malignant growth and their families.

National Cancer Institute (cancer.gov): A U.S. government organization with comprehensive information on cancer research, treatment, and clinical trials.

Remember to consult the most recent editions and updated resources to ensure you have the latest information. These resources can offer valuable insights, practical guidance, emotional support, and the latest developments in breast cancer care. By utilizing these references, you continue to enhance your ability to provide informed and compassionate support to your loved one on their breast cancer journey.

Conclusion

The Enduring Impact of Support: A Journey Shared

As the chapters of your loved one's breast cancer journey unfold, it's essential to recognize that the impact of your support extends far beyond the duration of treatments or recovery periods. This final note emphasizes the lasting significance of the support you've provided and the beautiful connection you've forged through shared experiences, resilience, and compassion.

A Bond Forged Through Challenges

Strength in Unity: Your unwavering presence, empathy, and understanding have strengthened your bond, creating a profound connection that transcends the challenges you've faced together.

Shared Moments: The shared moments of joy, laughter, and tears have woven a tapestry of memories that will be cherished for a lifetime.

The Ripple Effect of Compassion

Inspiring Others: Your dedication to providing support serves as an inspiration to others, showing the power of compassion and solidarity during difficult times.

Paying it Forward: The care and empathy you've shown will ripple outward, as your loved one may find themselves inspired to support others on their journeys.

Life Beyond Breast Cancer

A New Beginning: As your loved one moves forward, the resilience and positivity you've fostered will continue to shape their outlook on life, encouraging them to embrace each day with gratitude and hope.

Stronger Together: The challenges you've navigated together have forged a lasting connection, strengthening the foundation of your relationship and the love you share.

Continuing the Journey

An Ongoing Chapter: The journey you've shared during breast cancer has created a unique chapter in your relationship, one that will remain etched in your hearts as a testament to the strength of your bond.

Facing the Future: As you face the future together, remember the incredible impact you've had on each other's lives and the indomitable spirit that has carried you through.

A Heartfelt Thank You

Gratitude: Express your gratitude for the opportunity to be a part of this journey, for the lessons learned, and for the resilience that has grown from facing challenges together.

Enduring Connection: Embrace the enduring connection you've established, knowing that the love and support you've provided will always be a cherished part of your loved one's story.

In conclusion, the impact of your support is a gift that keeps on giving. Your compassion, strength, and unwavering presence have left an indelible mark on your loved one's breast cancer journey. As you move forward together, may you continue to cherish the shared moments, celebrate each triumph, and face the future with the enduring love and connection that have defined this remarkable chapter in both of your lives.